THE SLOW
SUBTRACTION

ALS

Joseph Powell

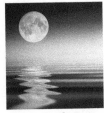

MoonPath Press

Poetry
ISBN 978-1-936657-48-3

Cover art by Beverly Ash Gilbert, *Break in the Storm*,
from the dreamy landscapes collection

Author photos by Rob Fraser

Book design by Tonya Namura
using Avenir Next Condensed and Gentium Basic

MoonPath Press is dedicated to publishing the
finest poets living in the U.S. Pacific Northwest.

MoonPath Press
PO Box 445
Tillamook, OR 97141

MoonPathPress@gmail.com

http://MoonPathPress.com

THE SLOW SUBTRACTION: A.L.S.

ACKNOWLEDGMENTS

I would like to thank the editors of the following magazines in which some of these poems were previously published, occasionally in slightly different versions. I would also like to thank Mark Halperin and Stephen Maurer for their suggestions and close reading of many of these poems. A special thanks to Alice Derry who gave this a thorough reading. I would also like to thank Central Washington University for its support of my work, and the National Endowment for the Arts whose grant gave me the time to complete many of these poems. Thanks also to Robert Bixby and March Street Press for publishing some of these poems in *Preamble to the Afterlife* in 2013.

Clover: "At Adrianne's House in Patmos"

Floating Bridge Review #5: "Kindness."

Homestead Review: "The Feeding Tube"

Weber—The Contemporary West: "The Flood," "The Slow Subtraction"

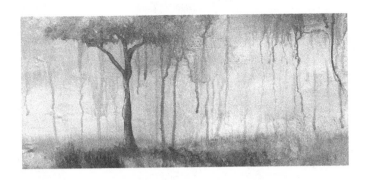

To Judith Kleck Powell
(1950-2012)

We scarce in thousands meet one kindred mind
And if the long-sought good at last we find
When least we fear it, death our treasure steals
And gives our heart a wound that nothing heals.

—John Milton, "The Death of Damon"

Contents

THE SLOW SUBTRACTION

ALS

I

A man who has nothing
can whistle in a robber's face.

—Juvenal, "Vanity of
Human Wishes"

HER DREAM

A red-haired woman dressed in sparkling
lights and a black gown steps on stage
with a kitchen chair, one hand shaping silence.

From the shadows behind her
leaps an immense black leopard with yellow eyes
who flows into the chair facing the audience.

The woman gives a signal.
The cat pads through the shadowed aisles, circling
the quiet crowd, closer and closer.

It slides into my wife's lap
as if she were the chair
or the leopard's mother
and whispers, "You're dead."

THE NEWS

The doctor's question is soft but direct.
"Well, do you think you have A.L.S.?"
He leans back in his chair, a pen to his lips,
his chamois shirt from L.L.Bean open at the collar,
sleeves rolled, ready.
"No. I don't think I do."

His pen moves to the other hand
as he sits up, "Well, I think you do."
He watches his news,
the crumpled face, tears,
hands covering so little.

The news dies on a dying tongue.
But comes back every morning after dreams.
It lives with the morning's coffee,
slurred words, the slurry of pills
dissolving all night in a cup of orange juice.
The first phone call, breakfast, hand-talking to the dog.

Doctors and nurses also remind her
of what's to come, speech machines,
the feeding tube, their storehouse
of spare parts for her use,
the tidy, civil commerce of the end.

Her hands still unfold the morning paper,
square as a window on the gang shootouts,
meth busts, bar knifings in Yakima.
Her story, not on any page
she can turn to, is always there
like the ash-print on her fingers.

FLOOD

We stood at the windows and watched
because there was so much else to do
and the water's rising was almost Biblical.
Eavesdropping on profligate power,
our lives seemed to twist up like windless smoke
not knowing how they'd scatter, dissolve.
The flood islanded us, a ten-foot stream on one side,
five feet on the other. Water seethed
through the trees, swallowing panels, beams,
tires, clots of wire and blue twine,
the way A.L.S. is taking your speech,
consonants and compounds of sound disappearing
like fenceposts or bridge timbers.

We stood marooned by sudden change
like the fascination of watching a snake,
its unhinged jaws stretching
around a squirrel, and pulse on pulse
the head, the shoulders, the chest,
disappearing until only the bushy tail
wags from its mouth, and we know
it's paralyzed inside
an incredible pulsing pressure.

Immensity has no government except its own motion,
forward, or back in eddies, its lawlessness a kind of reversal
in logic: trees bow down to strap on a harness of debris,
logs spin, and all that hurry and wildness,
aiming to spread into rest, into a lake
where burdens of silt will sift away.

Afterwards, everything left standing
wore a grass skirt. Tires leaned against fences
like juvenile smokers outside a tavern.

Barbed-wire had popped and lay across
the brow of the creek bank like stitches.
Horse turds hung in bare cottonwood branches,
a deer's body, a boa around a telephone pole.
Even the tatters seemed scrubbed clean,
the field shiny and raked like a lawn.
When you tried to speak, the words
had changed utterly, faltering and thick.
We could never look at the same world again.

BRIDAL SUITE

She seems as solid and hardy as the kitchen sink
where she performs her culinary voodoo,
yet the disease has climbed the staircase
of her brain, entered the bridal suite
and started to rip away the frilled curtains
with black leopard claws, letting the dark in,
stirring the dust of herself.

This diagnosis changes who she thinks she is,
like a wedding, whose groom knows her weaknesses
and can use them against her, but she rises
out of that closed room and begins to hum.

FAITH

She has passed through the heavy doors of grace.
Its spareness a kind of amplitude.
Small things wash away like bath water.
Even the choking for air after a bad swallow
has lost its wild-eyed reflex
as if she's stroking the leopard beside her
until breath comes back.

Her faith is in the rightness of demise,
in the mind's transformative evolution,
the feel of the enlarged pulse
in the sway of events, the way pettiness
is candleflicker against the passing night,
the divinity of sleep on cool afternoons.

She has taken the sacrament of faith
like a host into her failing body.
It enlightens the spiral of fragments
in memory's house—dust in sunlit rooms.
Love is the old dog asleep at the door.

BAKED CRAB STORY

After too much praise at dinner,
you tell the baked crab story again:
how in New Mexico, you never had seafood
so when uncleaned Dungeness crab
was brought home, you wrapped it in tinfoil
and baked it until the stink was unbearable
and had to be thrown out.

Now that you've perfected your culinary craft
and nothing is too large or small to master,
you were only showing how sour or plain
our first dishes are, that mistakes are success's ingredients,
a generous failing for all the non-chefs present.
Your story wanted to lead us back
to the joy of our pleasures,
our grunts and hums and closed-eye satisfactions,
not to be ruined by the spotlight of attention.

You forget it was your first husband, not me
who brought that crab home.
How anyone drew up this story like the wine
from their glasses in a sequence of stories
neither you nor I will ever know, just a daisy-chain
of things in language that shine, wilt, and darken.
But for me, the story, too, is an emblem
of how in memory's heaped-up library
we have become each other's narratives,
both text and footnote,
and how, now, our stories will soon be changed,
cut off from their dual legacy of facts.
They'll be like blown candles,
and drift off like interwoven smoke.

IRONIES

Her rich, efficient, assuring
crisis-line voice
is the first casualty.

⌒

Her thousand cookbooks
bore her off to sleep each night.
Her food believed in joy.
Now, she can't swallow.

⌒

"Oh, you look sooo good,"
friends who haven't seen her say
and squeeze their relief into a hug:
slenderness as beauty,
not death's throat-grip.

⌒

Like Cezanne coloring contour
with the smallest shades,
the twitching muscles remodel her face
which seems more peaceful, carefree.

⌒

She is learning to read us—our embraces,
our dismissals, our letters and notes—
the way God must
in His silence, His ineffable remove.

⌒

She photographs a goat's tracks in the wet sand
of Psilli Amo, pleased with leisure,
the beach to herself at the end of October.
Then notices her own footprints,
that thin line her right toe drags in the sand.

PARIS IN OCTOBER

I'll die in Paris in the pouring rain
a day I have a memory of already.
—César Vallejo

After the death news and the time it takes
to absorb it, we leave for Paris
as a refusal of the disease's black flag,
though it already makes every stair two.

Each morning we go to mass at Notre Dame,
take the host on hopeful tongues,
then walk to the Louvre, by outdoor shops,
flower and book stalls, along the constrained Seine
glassily forgiving its boats and plastic bottles.

Arm in arm, our slow progress
makes time our hostage. The plane trees drop
sequins from their yellow dresses onto the grass and gravel.
Red squirrels molting to grey
stop with a mouthful of seeds to watch our progress,
then leap into a litter of leaves.

Her deepest pleasure comes after two hours
of looking at deathless paintings and sculptures,
as she sits in the Louvre shop, writing
postcards, sipping coffee, Paris in her pen,
her hand still innocent of its own exile,
her loneliness reaching out to friends an ocean away.

TRAVELING

My being almost languageless in Greece echoes yours—
fingers are tongues, silence, a quality
in time and space, no olive for its branches.

A smiling face feels like a handshake.
Every suncurled cat knows
that distance is the soul's drug—
its languors, its sunlight, its peace.

Voices stream by and you float on that water
learning the properties of neglect,
the preamble to the afterlife.

            ∽

Last night we opened the upstairs door
to let the breeze into a hot night.
The curtains filled and luffed.
We read in bed till nearly midnight,
the taverna songs from Aloni
rising to the window, dancing inside.
They speak of another era, a death lament
about lives too true and large to lose.

            ∽

Through the upstairs door
a cat padded down the steep echoing stairs.
It tipped the garbage can,
spread out the trash. Sleeping late,
we heard nothing.
It found a lamb bone,
dragged it across the room, licked the marrow
till the white shone like ivory,
left footprints in the coffee grounds.

Black cat, I've seen you in that olive tree
behind the house where no one lives,
watching us and every passerby.
We have fed you almost all our lives.
You will have to wait outside.
Your time will come soon enough.

AT ADRIANNE'S HOUSE ON PATMOS

The lemon trees curl inward
and the warmth is a soft net over us,
a cloud so full of itself
it's about to rain, pulsing its blue
shadows across the evening.
The musk of our bodies, the earth
tensing with the thought of rain.

What's knowledge against this?
A cat creeps toward the night.
Moonlight will ignite its eyeteeth
and shine the lemons. A still lizard
watches from a crevice in the whitewashed wall.
We wait for the word, the weight
that will alter the tense balance,
for a lemon to release its purchase,
the lizard to flinch, for the cloudburst.

Everything we love about each other
over these last decades
climbs like the light up this tree,
until the fragrant dark enters us
the way we've entered each other,
and the book sits on its wings,
the cup in its saucer,
the shoe's tongue loosened.

THE FLU

Last night I ran to your choking and coughing
downstairs. "I'm sick," you squeezed out—
sickness had made your Sickness reel—
you gagged and sweated and trembled
in the kitchen without the lights on
over a plastic yellow washtub.

"I'll be okay, go to bed," each syllable
wrung out of that sponge in your mouth.

I brought a damp towel and left a corner light on.
Then lay in my own dark, listening—
footprints through my coffee grounds.

LIP

Trying to eat, you've bitten yourself
so many times a bruised knot
builds behind your lower lip
and you wad a napkin there
just to put some soft distance
between the pain and its nail.

Napkin wads are cast blossoms
like Gretel crumbs
wherever you go.

The witch bakes another plum shingle
and polishes her oven.

II

Order, but a still-life of chaos.

—Chris Hansen, "The Dark
Cloaked Figure"

IN BED, PAST MIDNIGHT

You type on your iPhone that you're afraid
of the feeding tube, how absolute it is.
You type each character
and the phone's face glows in the dark
making clicks like scales
of a turning snake if we amplified them
the way each thing in our lives is amplified now.

Your mother is staying with us
and you're frustrated by her memory,
lost purses and appointments,
the trauma of small changes.
You're mothering your mother
who clings, afraid for both of you.

Between each sentence, each message,
I listen to dog snores by the door,
the heater fan whirring,
the cat paws nicking along the hallway floor,
thin peepholes of sound away in the dark.

Here in this bed our child first
squiggled into life, candlelight burned
on our own assurances, and Marvin Gaye blessed
those nights we journeyed into each other.
It is the place our son's dread crawled to,
where thousands of books carried us off
to distant lands and lives like ours now.

Your changing body changes yet again,
the tube like the tag on a shirt you can't take off,
one less side to sleep on, one less, one less.

INTIMACY

As I wash your body with a fluffy yellow
ball of cloth squirted with liquid lavender soap,
going over your back, across your neck and face,
between and under each breast, down your legs
and feet, your butt and crotch, or shampooing your hair,
I'm caressing each mortal zone
with an embalming scent

yet this slow waltz we do from chair to bed
or car to chair or chair to chair
is more dancing than our busy lifetimes ever let us do.
With your arms around my neck,
feet like twisted paddles on oarlike legs,
head pressed against my chest,
we dance the fatal dance of our time's demise,
doubtless, fretless, as double-helixed as our son.

THE BLACK RABBIT

At four, our son is full of glee about the young rabbit
from his babysitter. He hops and claps
and wants to hold it. It sits inside itself
hugging its black coat, ears laid back,
nose twitching cautiously. We don't have a hutch
so it's in a cardboard box beside the shelves
of cookbooks in the kitchen.
He picks it up. We help him hold it.

All afternoon, I work at framing and nailing,
cutting chickenwire, stapling. It's dark before I finish.
Inside, we water and feed the rabbit,
but when a cookbook falls from the shelf
onto the tiled floor, the rabbit leaps
straight up and flips backwards,
its eyes bulging, feet scratching air.

When I lead my son to the box,
the rabbit was warm and limp, eyes blinkless.
He keeps trying to make it sit up,
to wake it with kindness.
When I explained it's dead,
he still pets it, watching it fall each time.

Now, as he bathes his mother
I think of that black rabbit,
my son righting it, two hours through his tears.
How he washes her carefully,
under the arms, shampooing her hair,
then the drying and dressing.

KINDNESS

Before we entered this phase
where death came barring every door,
human motive had a darker hue—
kindness seemed a pressure to accept
some negligence, some ancient injury
too scarred over to see at first, and so we looked.
Seeing deeply meant tracing how far suspicion went.

Yet with nothing to gain,
our friends come with lasagna,
roast beef, wine and bread, offers to clean the house,
make blankets and scarves, to stitch time
back into that cloth our lives have woven.

Many call, now, just to lighten that shadow at the door,
to make its shade step back into a deeper shade.
Though we mostly live and die in private,
tending like hens our clutch of pain,
leaving's hardest when spring comes
bustling in like a puppy,
and the mask by which we masked the world
drops off to reveal what was almost always there—
a hand outstretched in giving, without receiving,
and love for the love it's losing.

LATE BLOOMERS

By mid-July all the wildflowers have dried
and blown away. The sun, a red hot skillet.
Yet along the river canyon, up the arid ravines,
in crevices of rocky steppe
mock orange blooms in soil so parched
dust can't remember its name,
mobbed with blooms in half-scents of jasmine and orange.
Think of the reservoirs of stubborn commitment
in each branch, transforming adversity into such delicacy.
Blind Homer grinding out hexameters
in the cicada buzz and the still, olive heat of afternoons,
thousands of petals shaped from his parched sod.
Or late Yeats: out of the rubble of his dreams
and obligations to his country's past
he became the vicar of old age, a bitter sorrow
tending beauty's lonely church.
How Billie Holiday made pain so personal
all the back doors opened into coffins of alley light.
She's the night's ambassador, the desert's late flower.
Your disease has forged a witty courageous voice.
Perhaps adversity is that ground
on which we're broken or made new.
Your sure fatal syllables enlarge
like the sweet lather of petals in my hands.

THE SLOW SUBTRACTION

See what a beautiful thing a finger is,
see how much you ignored it till now.
Little digits who found music, sculpted,
drew in the dirt, held the oblong wonder of an egg.
They paid the bills, the heart's taxes, achieved
the opulence in the skin's sweet torment,
prayed, found the thousand graspable things.
They are the brain's viceroys of this new country.

When the left hand goes, so do olive lids
and gin caps, all slicing and dicing.
With the right hand, scissors, zippers, buttons,
toothbrushes, music, scratching itches. . .

What a dancer the wrist is, the arm's waist,
part labor, part juju, connoisseur of castanets.
It guided love into its cool embrace;
it unlocked doors, it believed in hope,
how things turn and turn on themselves
until that almost soundless click and release.
It was always among the first to say goodbye.

When the left leg loses its grip,
the world slows to a crawl.
It used to believe in leaving, the distances it crossed,
so this slowness is like the solidity of belief.
When the right leg goes,
and the feet twist to a soleless print,
muscles screwed tight as canning lids,
there is an exodus of shoes.
The walker, the canes, too, depart,
and all you stood for or could stand.

The body teaches its crash course
with example after tedious example,
until you lie there wondering what life might have been
had you loved each lost thing this much.

BACHELOR PARTY

She doesn't want me to leave, not even for a day.

You'll have plenty of time for it, when I'm dead,
imagining tasseled breasts, cake jumping,
some drunken groping.

I explain we're college friends with an excuse
to gather, all in our sixties. It's dinner and toasts,
no women at his house except three old teachers
catering through the summer.

Liar.
I know that against our best intentions
we're all liars bending stories to fit what we feel,
until truth is only what God knows.
In God's eye a prayer must be like a golden mote of dust
that rises from a garden, hemisphere, an era.
Her edged accusation is just another prayer,
a cloud to the Cloud, to that old sky
under which we used to live.

I do relish the womanlessness, the ease of it,
that change in verbal manners, the teachers speechless.
There is little truth we can count on, even God's.

Custom is the jaded matrix
we see by, not through.
We use it as we use each other,
and how cunningly crude we can be
when broken and angry.
How firmly, desperately, we hold on
to the ones we love.

WEDDING

My son and I dress her for a nephew's wedding
at the Party Barn on Stuart Anderson's old ranch.
She had the habit of buying expensive clothes
from second-hand stores she might someday wear,
though now she's dropped several sizes
below the thinnest she might imagine squeezing into.
We try the gold lamé, the green silk evening gown,
the neckless, backless, sleeveless,
then several different plain and floral shawls,
gold earrings, bracelets, a row of shoes,
then make-up, and blow-dried hair.
In her wheelchair, she says, "I feel like a queen,"
and laughs both at pampered pleasure and this irony.
Her fun is also the many choices,
a little glamour on a windless summer day,
her awkward male coiffeurs, this caesura in trouble's feast.

The parking lot is a mowed field, paths bark and gravel,
but we make our bumpy way to the ceremony
and sit beside a row of white chairs on a green lawn.
The usual petals, lacy trains, pronouncements
of love, for richer or poorer, in sickness and in health,
with Taneum Creek's half music in the background.
Wheeling back to the reception area, she begins to cry,
and the sound swells into an awful sob
all the language she's been left,
a wretched guttural requiem.

So we bounce our way back across the field,
leaving a trail of dust in the July afternoon,
a few sobs like fall colors in the heat-struck trees.
When the doctor called it *emotional incontinence*,
she asked, "should I wear a diaper on my head?"

Her humor saves much but covers little
like that empty space she sees in the future wedding
of our son, which widens into a grief she can't contain.

BIG PINES IN REAL TIME

Each hour is mixing and blending
and straining food for the P.E.G.,
washing and dressing, socking a foot
or unsocking it by the pellet stove,
with winter peering inside. The birds
at the feeder chase each other,
effortlessly, playfully mobile.

The day is gray with spots of light,
a few weightless snowflakes
like tinkling bell-sounds in the sun-struck air.
She can't move anything now
but inertia has its own restless energy
so I bundle her up,
get the wheelchair in the van,
and drive into the Yakima canyon.

Deer look up, then keep on eating.
On a dead tree branch, an eagle
sits inside herself like a hand in a muff.
Nothing in the landscape judges us.
We stop at Big Pines for its paved
walkways beside the river.

My hand on the joy stick,
we make tentative tracks in the faint snow.
No one is here. I jog along the campsite road.
The snowy wheels rooster-tail.
The green sun is tangled in needles.
A few leaves, yellow hearts snagged on cottonwoods.
The bed-ridden river rolling,
hurrying somewhere unknown to itself.

Then I run, spinning her
through space, motion swelling inside her
like real time. Her cap tilts above the smallest smile
her face can muster, the cold streams from her eyes,
her cheeks blush.

Even inside her cage, she is a bird,
fluttering invisible wings, flying.

WINTER RAINBOW

After days of rain and snow,
constant news of war and dying,
you stopped, pointed at the rainbow,
and said, *the green shined through*

among bands of yellow and red,
of violet and blue in a cold sky.
Your voice had lost its usual dread,
its calm warmth was a hunger fed.

You knew the planes of color dissolve,
that any joy's a passer-by,
but you sat, clearly satisfied
with light's refractive interval

as if some hope were a spectral color,
your favorite green, in winter weather.

IRONIES

She's in her wheelchair,
ramps on every step, yet frets
about the commode on the deck.

～

For four years we've prayed
for remission.
Now we pray it doesn't come.

～

It's true—
death climbing the ladder inside her
has a certain radiance.

～

The leopard has lain
a long time
with the lamb.

～

Many, many depletions,
enough to make
calm courage cry.

～

We never think of coughing
as a blessing
until we can't cough.

～

When you are dying
death is everywhere,
flippant, in all its cheapest forms.

YAKIMA CANYON IN WINTER

The dark comes early in this canyon
as we linger in the lateness of the afternoon,
sunlit, taking all these last colors in.
How striking the naked world is:
rosebush canes are clumps of frosted magenta,
leafless river willows, masses of tousled orange hair;
the bunchgrass glows. Like cold-darkened minds,
ponderosa pines rise elegantly on auburn stems.

A studious winter light magnifies the afternoon
and a stillness opens. Clusters of aspen spines
on the shady side of the canyon
are white rows of sunlicked candlesticks.
Each thing refuses to go down quietly,
believes in nuance, irrepressible essences,
change blossoming into change.

DEPENDENCY

When part after part after part is paralyzed
we retreat to the poverty of our needs.
Love is the burden and the burdened;
it's the who-you-were overlaid by the now-you,
memory of that mind sailing
so gracefully its wind-whipped seas;
it's those sensuous syllables of your inner ear
that made language curl so surely into itself;
it's the wreckage of the self to hear it again,
to ease the thousand humiliations—
a crackled cry for a voice, muscles deaf,
body swaddled by someone else;
it's our photo gallery of lost events
we've gone through one by one,
our images modeled into shapes
youth could never have imagined,
into that infant of our infancy;
it's the choking dread of the "paralytic
stunned in the tub and the water rising";
it's the joy of the moment inflamed
by the immanence of the next change,
by the thousand days of epilogue,
by the light-tossed world outside the window
the magnitude of its departure;
it's the beauty of your changing face,
that light inside your eyes
shining through your disbelief;
it's that pleasure in controlling
one's space *in absentia*—
that cruelty towards all we've lost
which is itself a kind of love.

PERSON

"She" is already trying to die,
to turn you into someone else.
She is the pictures on my walls, in my office,
the patient, the news I give our friends who ask.

You is for talking to you,
my second person, my second self.
Thirty-six years of "What do you think...."
"How would you...."
It is the person you are
inside my head.

You speak when I speak,
think what I think,
you're the Aegean to my island,
the sidewalks of my streets,
the door to my house, the house...

Inside my head, you are the person
who can never die.

Death's credence comes to us
in small costs, mounting and mounting.

—Ivan Doig, *Searunners*

JOURNAL EXCERPTS

§: Ice & Fire

Death begins to spin its wintry images: a dormant garden is a blank open book, a hawk in the cottonwood watches the river's edges slowly freeze toward the center.

We think of the intuitive grace of old animals who wander off from the herd and die, but your wandering off will take five years, and in that time our minds tour the past, climb into the future, and sit in surreal judgment over the present. The disease is pushing you farther and farther inward because outwardly people see you as someone they must talk louder to.

Each day you go to mass at St. Andrew's, to Starbucks for an iced four shots with heavy cream, work at the Food Bank, home. You fix something to eat and sit at a computer game called Bookworm. Red letters fall from the top of the screen, and you scoop up words before they burn.

§: Striped Lines

We drive to Mountain High Sports to get a Christmas
present for our son, a headlamp for cross-country
skiing. We park in a handicapped slot across the
street. I push the button on the van's dash to open the
side door and let the ramp slide out. At that moment
someone pulls into the yellow-striped area. Our ramp
hits his front wheel, trembles, draws back in, the door
closes, and the hydraulics underneath start a wild
knocking like someone with a hammer wants out, as
if winter has a real fist. On the door panel is a sticker
for Kelsey's, who installed the mechanism, a company
in Sumner. Someone tells me to take the battery cable
off the negative post. I have no tools. Meanwhile, the
banging continues, and you're locked in like a cat in
a large can. I run into Mountain High, and the owner,
Tammy, is talking to a customer. I wait. The pounding
resounds inside my head. Finally, she is done but has
only a pair of pliers. Just as I start to pry the cable off,
the knocking stops. I press the button and the ramp
slides out the way it's supposed to. Some snow was
piled in the handicapped area and half of the lines
are hard to see. But the driver never did see, or pay
attention to the ramp coming out.

Most of us don't read the striped lines, or the text
between them. To us, it's wasted parking space.
Montaigne says "everything that comes to our eyes
is book enough; a page's prank, a servant's blunder, a
remark at table, are so many new materials," yet what
we read, mostly, is our own needs, in the way we're
used to seeing and feeling them. By *page* he meant
a court's errand boy, but we could read the text of
striped asphalt, a strapped-in look, the tone of a ramp
extending.

§: Simple Pleasures

Evan takes you to a movie, but the battery connection on the chair pops loose, and the ramp is frozen—snow and ice clogged the mechanism. He drives you back home, but we can't get you out of the car. We have to borrow a manual wheelchair, and ease you out the front door and into the house. From the cold, your chin is trembling. We finally get you beside the fire. I take the chair apart and tighten and duct-tape the battery connections. Make a reservation to fix the ramp. The next day is warmer; on the way to town, I swerve into several ice bumps. When I stop, the ramp works fine. I cancel the appointment. But all winter, the only movie we see is the one we are in.

§: Wipers

I stop at Matheus Lumber to see my brother; it is
raining hard and I leave the wipers and radio and
motor on. When I come out ten minutes later, the rain
has slowed to a drizzle, and you've had to listen to the
screech of wipers going back and forth across a drying
window, as if a child with restless energy practiced a
violin inside your head. The promise of A.L.S. is like
being locked inside a van with squeaky wipers that
won't shut off. It's almost impossible to clear your
vision of persistent implacable facts. They beat their
way into your thinking again and again. You are stuck
inside, going nowhere, listening to the screech, screech,
screech of time's erasures.

§: Again & Again

About once a month it's the same. We are in Fred Meyer,
in a handicapped slot. When we get back to the car with
groceries, a jeep is parked in the cross-hatched section
so we can't let the ramp down and the wheelchair in.
It is Saturday afternoon. I have the store manager page
the jeep's owner, but he or she never comes out. Finally,
I back into traffic to let the ramp down. You feel like a
wreck in the road, the pause button in everyone's day.
New material.

§: Gassing Up

A woman in a Thunderbird at JR's Economart keeps
watching me, with the eye of a writer, as I give you
sips from a clear plastic cup, and dab your face to get
the dribbled water, then put a paper towel in your
mouth so saliva doesn't leak out. The woman's husband
is gassing up; she is watching raptly, a middle-aged
woman in a blue tailored dress with buttons up the
front. The watching is in genuine interest, a kind of
how-it's-done interest, curiosity about the infirm, but
pitiable too, as if she'd tell her bridge people about it,
her writing group. Glad, too, to have the windows and
space between us, to get a story about a woman with a
white paper blossom in her mouth.

§: Fusion

I wonder how much your requests for things—a
paper towel, clothing loosened, glasses cleaned,
lip gloss on, blanket over your knees, jello, an ear
scratch, a pillow adjustment—is a reassurance that
you're not powerless, that the little stone you have
left to flip into the water can still make a ripple, that
inner isolation has an outer world. Or if it is a kind
of dominance, like Marlin Barton's story in *The Best
American Short Stories*, 2011, where a mother smothers
her deaf daughter because she can't stand the special
attention she pays to the father, or the photographer
who comes to stay. Love's jealousy wants the beloved
near and nearer. It pulls her in like some larger star its
satellite, until its final form is fusion. The slide from a
fierce independence to complete dependence can be
anticipated but hardly imagined; anger and tears with
each loss—the movement of a foot, buttoning a sweater,
brushing teeth, cooking, walking, moving a hand to the
controllers on the wheelchair—until you are a body in a
chair. Maybe then you try to control those who control
your movement, time, comfort, sustenance, even your
distractions. Unable to speak clearly, you cry, shriek,
enter a kind of selflessness to assert the self. This
change, this new state, for each of us, is heavy and gives
off ungovernable heat.

§: Prison

You have entered fully the prison of your disease. You
can no longer move anything but your eyelids. You can
still eyetext, can still tell us what you need if you're
in front of the machine, but all other motion is gone.
We have a baby monitor on when you sleep, and you
can let out small urgent moans in desperate repetitive
sequences like the 19th Century Victorian mistress of
the house ringing her bell over and over, regardless of
how far the maid has to come or what she has to put
down. I'm often in the kitchen or at the computer or
reading in the study, three rooms away. It is hard not
to be annoyed by the sudden urgency, as if all other
urgencies are self-indulgence. What makes me turn
off the stove, save and exit, close the book, is that
thought of those cell doors, the ceiling you stare into,
that lovely frail flower inside your mind, still blooming.
Lowell wondered *Which is truer—the uncomfortable full
dress of words for print, or wordless conscious...no one ever
sees?* I doubt we're ever wordless; each word has its own
wardrobe, dressed up or down, even if it begins and
ends in silence.

§: Time's Weather

Every thing takes so much time: getting you up to pee
(out of the bed, into the electric wheelchair, into the
bathroom, onto the toilet, back into the chair, and into
the bed), back up to shower, to dress, then to get your
food ready for the P.E.G. The smallest tasks sit inside an
hour like a stone Buddha, a minute hovers like a fogbound
plane, an afternoon is a mountaintop miles away.

For you, loss is prologue to loss, and under-fixed in every
good, in every mood, is subtraction's next move. Time
speeds up. Blossoms move out from buds in rapid ecstasy,
then shrink and wither, each sentence ballooned and
italicized floats away dangling its length of string; the
leg, the arm, the hand fall like successive grains of sand,
and your face reflects that rose of evening when the hills
magnify, tensing for the crescendo when dark descends.

§: Letters

Many of your friends and old students send beautiful,
heartfelt tributes to your character, generosity, the
gift cooking gave them, your hospitality, your writing,
your courageous spirit. Each sends you into a seizure
of crying. You know you have three months, but your
mind refuses to comprehend it, and these tributes
contain the ache of all that living lost, ahead and
behind, the terrible finitude of love and beauty, the
scattering of your things and affections into some
inconceivable void. "I'm tired of being brave so others
can feel good," you eyetext one day. And you let the
letters pile up, until one afternoon when you're ready,
and feel strong enough, to cry.

§: Ringing

You finger the things you love—

the carnelian arrowhead found in the garden,
the painted floral plate she brought in Greece,
the cinnabar snuffbottle she bought with her own
necklace (yellow jade squash on one side,
the green of leaves on the other),
books like friends who never let you down—

all the while the phone is ringing
with Death's caller ID.

§: Eyetexts

You type on your eyetext machine: "I should stop
eating." Two days later, you are so weak you can't
eyetext anymore; your head bobs and you can't quite
move the letters from the keyboard to the text window.
You try valiantly to get out "all meds," to say you
want all your nightly meds, not just morphine. We
give you morphine four times a day, a little water to
get some of the other meds down: the anti-nausea pill
(prochlorperazine); the restless leg pill (gabapentin);
the anti-anxiety pill to help you sleep (lorazepam);
another pill to help you sleep (amitriptyline)). We crush
and dilute them to put them down your tube.

We have long looks of Icantbelievethisishappening,
a pleading wish to have this cup pass from us, of a
drowning person trying to get to the surface and
breathe. Your last eye-words are "all meds," but inside,
what trapped sentences ripple like wind-whipped silk?

IV

Death
begins the second time
with survival

—W.S. Merwin,
"The Second Time"

THE FIFTH NIGHT

Without food or water, the nurse says,
it takes about a week to die.
Two days left, my wife lapses into unconsciousness:
a faint lip quiver and a radiant bed-heat
as if her body struggled even harder
against the brain's cannibal neurology,
its strict machine persistence.

Outside, dark assembles itself
at all the windows and door-panes
like a brass band, death's saints,
waiting for orders to come marching in.
As I lie beside her, I read the walls,
the green flowery swirls in the paper,
the borders unglued in the tight spots.
The whole house seems at the bottom
of a vortex. I stand to breathe,
readjust her covers, exposing one foot
the way she likes it.

I take a blanket from the closet, my pillow,
and lie on the floor with the dog.
Afraid of the quiet inside her nightgown,
the hot labor of her dying,
I want to lie down with the living,
with the loyal future and its old ease,
the hard floor, a penance for survival.

The dog thinks I have come down to play.
I hold her firmly, to quiet her,
to lean into her fur blanket,
but she won't or can't hold still.

I get up, walk the dark house, turning on lights.
Outside, no red moon in the sky, no falling star,
so I return to bed, to face the music.

PERMISSION

Unconscious for over twenty-four hours,
she lay in her own shroud of heat
still as the death she must embrace.
Her body was in its third great labor.
In this war, the spirit hung on,
the body too using whatever slender weapons
it could marshal against death's grip.
We stood by, helplessly helping:
turning the covers, adjusting her body, soft music,
talking and stroking her hair and cheek.
When her father died four years before
she had called this "the hardest work we do."

To the hospice nurse, we described
this stand-off, her body's inert determined stasis,
how long it went on. At the door, leaving, the nurse asked
whether I'd given her "permission to die,
to move on. She might be waiting for that."
Improbable as it seemed, tritely spiritual,
and sentimental for one so attuned to herself,
so resolved and unflinching in this journey,
I got on my knees and talked,
loving her, saying I'd take care of the children,
that it was okay to leave now.
For the first time in two days, she blinked,
opened her eyes and looked at me
as if straining to see, dragging herself awake,
into a knowing, comprehending look.
I held her hand and she closed her eyes again.
I left and her son went to her,
came back and said, "she's gone."

The nurse said hearing is our last sense to leave,
but why is it we need permission to go?
Maybe the mind's long fight, day after day,
to push open the doors of consciousness,
habit's awesome urge to push through veils
and veils of grayness going dark.
Is love so needy to the last that its final touch
wants touch to reassure its journey,
like an only child stepping on its first bus to school?

I imagined her standing before the unknown,
its mysterious teacher beside the blackboard.
So new, she's not prepared to enter this room,
all those eons of souls already there.
Noiselessly, I want to take her hand,
walk her to the tiny seat among the truly dead.

GIFTS

At Christmas, I worried what to buy—
we knew her dying was weeks or months away.
She said she wanted nothing,
that nothing was her next inheritance,
an everlasting gift
her humor darkened by its truth.

I bought the softest full-length flannel nightgown
I could find, even the Peter Pan collar
was white and flecked with tiny roses.
With it maroon knee-high leg warmers
so she could sit beside the pellet-stove and watch the news.

Doesn't a gift hold out its promise
like an extended hand,
hope its parti-colored bow?
Doesn't its bright paper say *remember me?*
She had no hands to untie it,
unable to save the paper.

The beauty she beheld in her own dying—
how it trivialized those failures we're prone to rub,
found a way back to her estranged father,
revived a love for the silk of her syllables,
made the lit-up world step to the window and salute—
was her gift to me.

When the two men from Affordable Funeral Care
came in their blue ties and old overcoats
to take her body away on a black stretcher
like an athlete from her field of praise,
they had put on their best vacant solemnity,
a polite gum-chewing downcast silence,

but as they transported her,
I was grateful for that nightgown
so thinly protecting her last privacy,
for those few small pink roses sent
with her into the cold gloom of February.

THE FALLS

After five years of loss on loss,
we were inured to trauma, and one more announcement
was like St. Sebastian's eleventh arrow.
But when she eyetexted after her family's visit,
I should stop eating, each letter blinked out deliberately,
I took it, at first, with that numb finality we were used to.
Her bowels had shut down. Only her eyelids moved.

We sat watching the blackbirds fight at the feeder,
the colors on their shoulders like red eyes
against the new snow. Daffodils had emerged
on the sunny side of the house. So much was in readiness
to move on, and us holding back,
our ship anchored above the falls.

That night, I stopped giving her food and water
except to wash down the crushed pills and morphine.
It was like cutting the rope, starting the week-long drift.
Months later, I still shrink before that *should*.

MATES

Last winter, hunting season,
my brother and his wife looked for agates in Dry creek.
A wild Canada gander followed them,
honking, wing-flapping, charging, falling away.
He wouldn't be shooed,
and finally flew at my brother's wife,
his nails raking her shoulder,
wings whapping her head and hair,
attacking her back, again and again.
My brother broke its neck with a whirled stick.
Later, they found the body of its mate
face-down at the creek's edge.

I've seen the lone goose circle back
after its mate crumpled in the cornfield
from flying too close to the decoys,
shot in its fly-by worry.

Love can drive the self from hiding
and go down into its own labyrinth
with a mad flurry. I know the turns,
its blind alleys, false paths, and brief releases.

I too came back and back
to the one face-down in the creek
clawing at each fragile hope,
lost, with no one or thing to blame.
With no Ariadne, no string.

MATE ELEGY

A thin whirring in the grass.
At first just a moth trying to fly.
Then attached to its abdomen
his mashed, stepped-on mate.
His abdomen, too,
smashed into hers.

I pick him up, her body dangling
like the broken half of a flower.
Launched, he staggers through the air
some fifty feet
dragging her, his old joy,
her dead weight and memory,
aloft for as long as he can bear her
then sinks back into the grass.

WHITE SPACES

Dance the space between the steps; it is not stillness.
Hear the music between the notes; it is not silence.
Read the white between the lines; it's not empty.
             —Judith Kleck Powell, "Not Easy"

Where is it the spirit goes? At first so vast
you are every footstep's echo, and the night
has no corners, no exits. It's a map
with a living legend and names.
Then the steady erosions.

What remains of you shrinks to a weak beacon
on a fog-bound promontory, a light that rotates
with the seasons—birthdays and Christmases,
events we commemorated—or things I pick up
to dust, the picture of you and Joan in Greece.
And the dust on the rag, my hands,
that I inhale, as if time were a substance.

Other moments you come back quietly
unexpected: an unwritten thank-you note—
Dear Xemina, above a cluster of red zinnias
and blue bachelor buttons and all that white space,
the unfinished impulse, the gratitude that hangs
unsaid, floating somewhere between impulse and act.

What Porlock stole your words away?
What urgency—me, the phone, stove timer,
our dog's announcement of an arrival?
How easily, selflessly, you leant yourself
to some need knocking at our door.

For every word you left, an acre of white space
waits for your pen's touch.
Like a blank page, your silence
holds some pressing message, some promise,
as if I'm waiting for you to come,
pick up your pen, and fill it in,
as if there's unheard music in it,
some dance left inside the stillness.

A LETTER

We spent so much time together—
at work, home—there isn't one letter
to go back to in your sparse hand
(no cursive flourish, but a sliding print like stiff dancing).
I have your bouquet of poems, of course,
their charmed casual music
and that stark darkness only their sound could soothe.
Fearless, too, in the way they absorbed abuse—
taking those curses from a carload of delinquents
shouting down their own lives to anyone in earshot,
your brother's hand under the sheets, on his knees,
"dull saw seized in green wood," you wrote, the other hand
on a "budding breast" was a "swarm of bees on a bird's nest."
But a letter might tell of spaying the cat, a strange bone
in the yard, how dinner is tasteless eaten alone.
It needn't be polite. That bastard, the neighbor,
yelling at you for something I did.
His dog shitting on our grass again.
You were at your best with a martini
saluting smug ignorance like a relative
who'd just decided to shove off,
laughter like an extra olive in your glass, a bon voyage.
You were good at icepick epithets
that pinned old colleagues' faults
on the proverbial wall, playfully,
as if posted to an address in hell
where we'd all live like neighbors, eventually.
I miss your unflappable will
that tore toasters and mixers apart
to fix wiring, botched soldering, that broke horses,
trussed and dressed Julia's boneless duck,

your seven courses with different sorbet palate cleansers—
tongue serenades, mouth lullabies,
meals built like a love story's arc.

᷎

In your last two years
you looked death in the eye
and winked, gave him the finger
at all our lost time.
But I want that nerve, that wink.

I want that height
in your leap of faith

I want the way you read a horse—
a cocked ear or hoof, a bunched stillness,
its alphabet of breaths.

I want the smell of your neck—
like sandalwood and soap—
the way it lazed each line of my thought.

I miss your spices,
their cozy polylingual parties,
how they saved my soups, flat pastas,
rash experiments.

I want, again, the silence
we often travelled through—
inter-assured, avidly reading
the blessed world before us.

Your girlhood on the ranch in New Mexico
riding horses through pines and Indian relics,
dust, was soul-salve in every city or place we lit,
a rhythm like a heartbeat, the pulse of a musical sentence.
Sometimes your ranch world was the sweet melancholy
of exile; others, timelessness, where you watched
a shrike busily pinning potato bugs on strands
of barbed wire, its larder,
that first-time witness of a clever selfish cruelty,
raccoons crunching the shiver out of foot-long crawdads,
late summer fish gasping for air in the thinning creeks,
each beautiful and terrible thing in the world
resonating outward from this one.

You loved the smell of horse sweat and heat, that power
beneath you, at your command, and that childish dream
of setting out across the plains of grass and pine canyons
for some unattainable oasis, almost palpable
in its unreality, or something vulnerable to save,
a calf pinned in a hawthorn thicket,
an arrowed deer, a beautiful woman roped to the tracks,
then home again to the love of faces
ringed around pots of steam, glasses and silverware.
Some deep-seated, heartfelt illusion impossible to feign
or forget. You loved ristras thatched in straw
and hung on clotheslines, more beautiful to you
than that Minoan mosaic of the fisherman
with his string of red fish on my tee-shirt from Xania.
The green charcoal smell of chilies roasting in September,
turned over and over in their wire cages
on Albuquerque's streets
until that smell was dense as a sexual yearning—
warm, savory, intoxicating.

You brought a gunnysack of them back on the plane,
paying for the extra freight, wanting to bask in that smell,
to bring it home, to freeze that taste in time.

As I am frozen in this letter
both to you and about you
as death itself blurs this distinction.
I talk as if something deep inside split
some infinity and you could both answer and overhear.
Just this morning I opened a jar of jelly
you made and labeled "Tomato Jam: Fancy Pantry"
in your quick, leaning script, as tasty
as the jam with sausage. Labeled and label,
as proximate as nutshell and nut.
You, both so fully here and not.

TO AN UNBORN DAUGHTER

Now when your mother's dead
why do my thoughts turn to you so often,
the woman you might have been, her legacy.

And to the guilt of our (mostly my) need
as older parents to know your genes were clean,
and how horribly wrong that went.

She would say I never wanted you enough,
I, that life is skewed enough against us
not to want a fair and even field.

For years sorrow turned us from each other,
the *no* in every *yes*, the blown smoke
of birthday candles,
the olive at the bottom of the martini glass.
In her distress she named you
and died with it still inside her.

You arrive regularly like unopened letters
though you never posted a living word.
Your spirit roams an empty house.

A daughter's father-love can be eloquent.
With that elixir, she has turned
a man's-man—the pubster, hardhat, athlete—
into a doll-carrying, nail-painted, hand-holding
advocate of all things in her imagination.
He'll push her swing until she tires of it,
press her tears to his chest,
buy purple unicorns and silly polkadots.

Blood of blood, you would teach me a new innocence:
what I might dismiss in your mother
I'd embrace in you.

I've seen what that love can forgive,
the way she shaved his old face,
combed his hair, how her loyal grief,
vigilant, disturbs her sleep, her waking,
how it wheels him through the home's garden path
stopping for birds and flowers, soft words.
I'll get no such forgiveness.

But it's not your devotion
in some orbit around mine,
ours, that I want, but in all of grief's unravelings
to let your short life loose like a balloon,
clutched for decades,
to watch its wind-borne ascension,
the string waggling upward,
our breaths inside you so light
you rise and rise without us.

THE SNAKE

The summer after your death our trees
which most years were frosted and fruitless
bear loads I have to unburden.

Each room in the house is booby-trapped
with memories of half-lost joys.
So much fruit impossible to thin.

An imposed simplicity takes on the feeling
of an exile. Abandoned in an empty Eden,
I pick raspberries, blackcaps, blackberries

and freeze them on cookie sheets.
Bags and bags of fruit arranged like prisoners,
each guilty of untimely bounty.

Yet the yellow-striped garter snake coiled
in the leaves of the raspberry canes,
waiting for grasshoppers, seems right,
and the thin-waisted wasps I flick

off the ripe fruit. Trying to blend in,
I too wait in the green and yellow leaves,
wound inside a fading abundance,
arbiter of thorns, guardian of sweetness.

POSTHUMOUS DREAMING

In a dream, you, dream-like, slip away.
You wanted out, wherever *out* is, or what
cul-de-sac your love seemed trapped in, for silence
is the language of this unwaking, this restless
resting where you appear to disappear.
You're young again and beautiful, as if our thirty-six
years had traveled backward to its source,
that party where we found each other.
Now, you make fleeting, fleeing choices
through the many inner veils of my dream-light.
I can't keep up. You go further inside
my mind, then vanish as if by vanishing
you're more surely here, how waking's disturbed,
a morning lost to losing you, again.

DREAMS

One recurs. Sometimes I'm at a party,
a family gathering with a crowd of people.
I can't find you, but then some well-meaning friend
says you're here, but you don't want to see me.
I look from room to room and slowly get the news
you're leaving me, just moving on,
going back to New Mexico,
changing your life. More rooms, more people.
But no explanations. I see you once
in profile, by a window, young again exactly
like a favorite picture of you reading in a hammock.

The other came only once.
After a long time away, you return.
I look for you but you keep a cool distance,
hardly look at me until finally you're pressed to tell me
you're pregnant, but the child isn't mine.
I both do and don't want the child
but it's the way you speak to me
that disturbs. Take it or leave it,
the distance on your face says,
that firm way you plant the news.
Is death the child? Our daughter? Am I that child
waiting to separate from you, little astronaut
waiting to deboard the mother ship?

Both dreams contain a sequence of silences—
I search, but you hardly look my way.
You're young, beautiful, whole,
as if we're courting, as if our years didn't exist.
In each, you're uncommitted, free to roam
whichever way your wind blows
like a movie star with lots of money.
So unlike the often choiceless life

you thought you sometimes led,
or how the early choices, your parents' disapprovals,
hemmed you in, even the love we chose.

I see the mind's improbable demise
creating its own child, its own world
to fix the blasted world it lived in.
Awake, I feel betrayed, but want you free,
that child in you that was never mine to love.

Notes

1. In "Dependency" I use a quotation from Roethke's "The Meadow Mouse," found in *The Collected Poems of Theodore Roethke*, p. 219.
2. The P.E.G. referred to in several poems is an acronym for percutaneous endoscopic gastronomy which is a tube that has been surgically implanted into the stomach to feed patients when swallowing is impossible.
3. The epigraph by César Vallejo in "Paris in October" comes from Geoffrey Brock's translation in "Exhuming Vallejo" published in *Poetry*.
4. In the "Striped Lines" section of "Journal Excerpts," the Montaigne quotation comes from "Of the Education of Children," published in *Selections from the Essays*, ed. by Donald M. Frame, p. 15.
5. In the "Prison" section of "Journal Excerpts," the Robert Lowell quotation comes from the "No Telling" section of "Leaving America for England," in *Dolphin*, p.67.

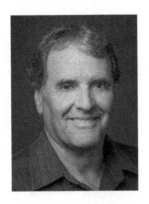

ABOUT THE AUTHOR

Joseph Powell was born and raised in Ellensburg where he worked hauling hay, digging ditches, and cultivating corn. Inspired by dirt and sweat, he received degrees from the University of Washington, Central Washington University, and his MFA from the University of Arizona. He met Judith Kleck in a graduate English class at Central Washington University, and they became life-long companions. After teaching high school at Sequim for a year, he decided only the tough and the brave could put up with those demands, so he applied for a job at Central Washington University.

He has published six collections of poetry: *Counting the Change*, which won the Quarterly Review of Literature's Book Award in 1986; *Winter Insomnia*, which was published by Arrowood Books in 1993; *Getting Here*, which also won the Quarterly Review of Literature's Book Award in 1997. Two books, *Hard Earth* (2010) and *Preamble to the Afterlife* (2013), were published by March Street Press. *Holding Nothing Back* was published by Main Street Rag in 2019. His book of short stories, *Fish Grooming & Other Stories*, was a finalist for the Washington State Book Award in 2008. He has also co-written a book on poetic meter with Mark Halperin called *Accent on Meter*, published by NCTE in 2004. For his poetry he has won a National Endowment for the Arts Award (2009), an Artist Trust award (2005), the Tom Pier Award (2006), and eleven poems have been nominated for Pushcart prizes from ten literary magazines. An essay won the Victor J. Emmett, Jr. Memorial Award from *The Midwest Quarterly* (2007). He has been Central Washington University's Phi Beta Kappa Scholar of the Year (2004), and was awarded Distinguished University Professor in Artistic Accomplishment (2009).

He taught in the English department at Central Washington University for thirty years. He lives on a small farm outside Ellensburg and is an avid gardener, flyfisherman, and scrounge—hunting mushrooms and agates, picking berries.